COMPLETE CRAVINGS

INTERMITTENT FASTING

FOR WOMEN OVER

40

Craving Slow Aging And Promoting Mental Clarity Through A Detoxifying Intermittent Lifestyle, Also Enhancing Metabolism For The Body Healings.

MOH LIMS

Copyright © 2023 by Moh Lims

TABLE OF CONTENT

INTRODUCTION

Complete Cravings Intermittent fasting for Women Over 40 is a deliberate eating program aimed at promoting general health, well-being, and weight management in a holistic and age-appropriate manner.

Maintaining a balanced and healthy lifestyle becomes even more important for women in their forties and beyond. Intermittent fasting, or a regulated eating routine, can be an effective method for reaching these objectives.

This collection of 20 expertly picked dishes is intended to support ladies over the age of 40 on their intermittent fasting journey. Each recipe includes a carefully chosen set of components that not only meet nutritional requirements but also satisfy the taste buds.

These recipes are nutrient-dense, filling, and varied, making fasting a fun and sustainable exercise.

Furthermore, in addition to the delectable aromas and gastronomic sensations provided by these recipes, each recipe is accompanied by its own set of health advantages and practical applications.

It's not just about cutting calories; it's about optimizing nutritional intake, boosting energy levels, and delivering the sustenance that women in this age group require.

Join us on this trip to explore how Complete Cravings Intermittent Fasting can be a tasty and purposeful approach for women over 40 to embrace a healthier, more vibrant existence.

1: Green Smoothie

Ingredients:

- 1 cup spinach

- 1/2 cucumber

- 1/2 avocado

- 1 cup coconut water

- 1 tbsp chia seeds

Instructions:

1. In a blender, combine the spinach, cucumber, avocado, coconut water, and chia seeds.

2. Blend until the mixture is smooth and creamy.

3. Serve in a glass as a nutritious breakfast throughout your eating window.

Benefits:

• High in vitamins and minerals

• Aids in weight management

• Hydrating and refreshing

Application:

• Eat throughout your eating window as a breakfast choice.

2: Greek Quinoa Salad

Ingredients:

- 1 cup cooked quinoa
- 1/2 cup cherry tomatoes
- 1/4 cup diced cucumber
- 1/4 cup feta cheese
- 2 tbsp olive oil
- 1 tbsp lemon juice
- Fresh oregano

Instructions:

1. Combine cooked quinoa, cherry tomatoes, chopped cucumber, and crumbled feta cheese in a large mixing basin.

2. Drizzle with olive oil and lemon juice, followed by fresh oregano.

3. Combine the ingredients and serve as a filling lunch or dinner choice throughout your eating window.

Benefits:

- High in fiber and protein, Beneficial to digestive health and Promotes fullness

Application:

• Ideal for a light lunch or dinner throughout your eating window.

3: Zucchini Noodles with Pesto

Ingredients:

- 2 medium zucchinis, spiralized
- 1/4 cup basil pesto
- Cherry tomatoes
- Pine nuts

Instructions:

1. Spiralize zucchini to make "zoodles."

2. Toss the zoodles with the basil pesto and serve with the cherry tomatoes and pine nuts on top.

3. Use as a light and tasty meal during your eating window.

Benefits:

- Low in carbohydrates and calories
- High in healthy fats and nutrients
- Helps with weight loss

Application:

- A healthy and filling dinner option.

4: Berry Overnight Oats

Ingredients:

- 1/2 cup rolled oats

- 1/2 cup almond milk

- 1/4 cup mixed berries

- 1 tbsp honey

- Chia seeds

Instructions:

1. Combine rolled oats and almond milk in a jar.

2. Stir in the mixed berries, honey, and chia seeds.

3. Stir thoroughly, cover, and place in the refrigerator overnight.

4. Give it a good stir in the morning and serve as a substantial breakfast.

Benefits:

- High in fiber

- Aids in blood sugar regulation

- Improves heart health

Application:

- Serve as a hearty breakfast.

5: Salmon with Asparagus

Ingredients:

- 6 oz salmon fillet

- 1 bunch asparagus

- Olive oil

- Lemon

- Garlic

- Dill

Instructions:

1. Toss the salmon in a bowl with olive oil, lemon zest, garlic, and dill.

2. Bake at 375°F (190°C) for 15-20 minutes, or until the salmon flakes easily.

3. Serve with roasted asparagus for a nutritious and tasty dinner during your eating window.

Benefits:

• High in omega-3 fatty acids

• Promotes brain health and Strengthens bones

Application:

• A nutritious and delectable dinner option.

6: Egg and Vegetable Stir-Fry

Ingredients:

- 2 eggs
- Bell peppers
- Broccoli
- Snap peas
- Soy sauce
- Ginger

Instructions:

1. In a nonstick skillet, scramble the eggs.

2. Remove the eggs from the pan and stir-fry the bell peppers, broccoli, and snap peas.

3. Season with soy sauce and ginger.

4. Mix the eggs and vegetables together and serve as a nutritious lunch during your eating window.

Benefits:

- High protein content
- Increases metabolism
- Helps with muscle maintenance

Application:

- Perfect for a quick and healthy lunch.

7: Avocado and Chicken Wrap

Ingredients:

- Grilled chicken breast
- Whole-wheat tortilla
- Avocado slices
- Lettuce
- Greek yogurt sauce

Instructions:

1. Grill and slice the chicken breast.

2. Arrange avocado and lettuce on a whole-wheat tortilla.

3. Drizzle the Greek yogurt sauce over the cooked chicken.

4. Roll it up and serve as a filling lunch.

Benefits:

- Provides balanced macronutrients
- Promotes bone health
- Improves skin and hair quality

Application:

- A filling lunch option.

8: Butternut Squash Soup

Ingredients:

- 2 cups butternut squash, cubed

- 1 onion

- Vegetable broth

- Coconut milk

- Nutmeg

Instructions:

1. Saute cubed butternut squash and onions in a saucepan until tender.

2. Bring the vegetable broth to a boil, then reduce to a low heat and simmer until the squash is cooked.

3. Puree the ingredients, then add in the coconut milk and season with nutmeg.

4. Use during your dining window as a warm and nourishing meal.

Benefits:

• High in vitamins and antioxidants, Promotes immunological function and Aids digestion.

Application:

• A hearty and nourishing supper option.

9: Cucumber and Tuna Salad

Ingredients:

- Canned tuna

- Sliced cucumber

- Red onion

- Greek yogurt dressing

Instructions:

1. Combine canned tuna, sliced cucumber, and diced red onion in a mixing dish.

2. Drizzle with Greek yogurt dressing and toss to combine.

3. During your eating window, enjoy this light and refreshing salad as a filling meal.

Benefits:

- High in protein

- Low in calories

- Aids in hydration

Application:

- A light and energizing lunch.

10: Lentil and Vegetable Stew

Ingredients:

- Red lentils
- Carrots
- Celery
- Onion
- Vegetable broth
- Turmeric

Instructions:

1. In a pot, combine red lentils, diced carrots, celery, and onions.

2. Stir in the veggie broth and a pinch of turmeric.

3. Cook until the lentils and vegetables are soft.

4. During your eating window, serve this hearty stew as a healthful supper alternative.

Benefits:

- Excellent source of plant-based protein
- Promotes digestive health
- Increases metabolism

Application:

- Perfect for a hearty dinner.

11: Chocolate Protein Smoothie

Ingredients:

- 1 scoop chocolate protein powder
- 1 banana
- Almond milk
- Almond butter
- Cacao nibs

Instructions:

1. Combine a scoop of chocolate protein powder, a banana, almond milk, almond butter, and cacao nibs in a blender.

2. Puree until smooth, then serve as a post-workout snack or breakfast.

Benefits:

- High protein content
- Aids in muscle repair
- Satisfies sweet cravings

Application:

- A snack or breakfast alternative post-workout.

12: Spinach and Feta Stuffed Chicken Breast

Ingredients:

- Chicken breast
- Spinach
- Feta cheese
- Garlic
- Lemon zest

Instructions:

1. Stuff the chicken breast with fresh spinach and crumbled feta cheese.

2. Season with garlic and lemon zest to taste.

3. Bake for about 25-30 minutes at 375°F (190°C).

4. Serve as a tasty and protein-rich meal.

Benefits:

- High in protein
- Promotes bone health
- Increases satiety

Application:

- A filling and protein-rich dinner.

13: Chia Seed Pudding

Ingredients:

- Chia seeds
- Almond milk
- Berries
- Honey

Instructions:

1. In a jar or bowl, combine chia seeds and almond milk.

2. Stir in the mixed berries and honey.

3. Stir well, cover, and place in the refrigerator for several hours or overnight.

4. Serve as a nutritious breakfast or snack.

Benefits:

- High in fiber and antioxidants
- Promotes digestive health
- Increases energy

Application:

- A quick and healthful breakfast or snack.

14: Broccoli and Quinoa Bowl

Ingredients:

- Roasted broccoli
- Cooked quinoa
- Chickpeas
- Tahini dressing

Instructions:

1. Blend almonds and pitted dates in a food processor until the mixture turns sticky.

2. Pulse in a pinch of vanilla extract.

3. Make little energy bites out of the mixture.

4. Refrigerate and serve as a fast, on-the-go snack.

Benefits:

• High in fiber and plant-based protein

• Beneficial to digestive health and Helps with weight loss

Application:

• A healthy lunch or dinner option.

15: Almond and Date Energy Bites

Ingredients:

- Almonds

- Dates

- Chia seeds

- Vanilla extract

Instructions:

1. Blend almonds and pitted dates in a food processor until the mixture turns sticky.

2. Pulse in a pinch of vanilla extract.

3. Make little energy bites out of the mixture.

4. Refrigerate and serve as a fast, on-the-go snack.

Benefits:

- Natural energy boost

- High in fiber and healthy fats

- Satisfies sweet cravings

Application:

- Perfect for a fast on-the-go snack.

16: Stuffed Bell Peppers

Ingredients:

- Bell peppers
- Ground turkey
- Quinoa
- Black beans
- Tomato sauce

Instructions:

1. Remove the tops and seeds from the bell peppers.

2. Prepare the ground turkey and quinoa separately, then combine with the black beans and tomato sauce.

3. Stuff the peppers with the mixture and bake for 25-30 minutes at 350°F (175°C).

4. Consume as a filling dinner during your eating window.

Benefits:

• High in protein and fiber

• Aids in weight loss and Promotes heart health

Application:

• A filling dinner option.

17: Veggie Omelette

Ingredients:

- Eggs

- Bell peppers

- Spinach

- Tomatoes

- Cheese (optional)

Instructions:

1. Beat the eggs and throw them into a hot, oiled pan.

2. Stir in the diced bell peppers, spinach, tomatoes, and cheese (if using).

3. Continue to cook until the eggs are set.

4. Cut in half and serve as a nutritious breakfast or brunch choice.

Benefits:

- High in protein

- Helps with muscle maintenance

- Increases satiety

Application:

- A nutritious breakfast or brunch choice.

18: Cauliflower Rice Stir-Fry

Ingredients:

- Cauliflower rice
- Shrimp or tofu
- Mixed vegetables
- Soy sauce

Instructions:

1. Stir-fry cauliflower rice with shrimp or tofu and a veggie mixture.

2. Season with soy sauce.

3. Cook until everything is well heated.

4. Serve as a light and filling meal during your eating window.

Benefits:

- Low in carbohydrates and calories
- High in nutrients and Helps with weight loss

Application:

- A light and filling meal.

19: Blueberry and Almond Smoothie Bowl

Ingredients:

- Blueberries

- Almond milk

- Almond butter

- Granola

Instructions:

1. Combine blueberries, almond milk, almond butter, and a scoop of protein powder in a blender.

2. Transfer to a bowl and top with granola.

3. During your eating window, enjoy this visually beautiful and nutritional breakfast.

Benefits:

- High in antioxidants

- Promotes heart health

- Increases energy

Application:

- A visually stunning and filling breakfast.

20: Cinnamon Baked Apples

Ingredients:

- Apples
- Cinnamon
- Walnuts
- Greek yogurt (optional)

Instructions:

1. Peel and slice the apples.

2. Garnish with cinnamon and walnuts.

3. Serve with a dollop of Greek yogurt, if desired.

4. Bake for 20 minutes at 350°F (175°C).

5. Serve as a nutritious dessert or snack during your eating period.

Benefits:

- High in fiber and antioxidants
- Beneficial to digestive health
- Satisfies sweet cravings

Application:

- A nutritious dessert or snack.

CONCLUSION

Finally, the Complete Cravings Intermittent Fasting plan for Women Over 40 offers a one-of-a-kind opportunity to improve overall well-being through a well-structured, balanced, and purposeful approach to eating.

We looked at 20 exquisite meals, each carefully chosen to meet the nutritional demands and appetites of women in this age bracket. But it's more than simply a cookbook; it's a guide to a better, more lively way of living.

Our nutritional needs change as we age, and our bodies demand more attention. When combined with the correct ingredients and attentive eating practices, intermittent fasting can help women over 40 manage their weight, increase energy levels, and promote a slew of health advantages.

The road to increased health and vitality is a personal one, and these recipes will help you along the way. Whether you incorporate them into your daily routine or simply draw inspiration from them, remember that taking charge of your nutrition is a powerful step toward a healthier, happier self.

Accept the Complete Cravings Intermittent Fasting diet as a versatile tool in your quest for wellness, and experience the delectable pleasures of a healthier, more fulfilling existence.